Cancer and Me

Cancer and Me

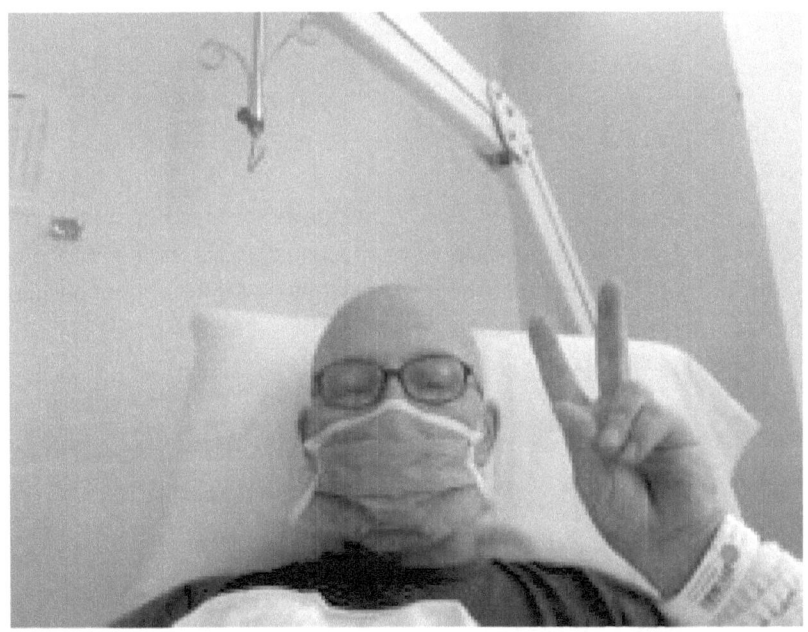

MICHAEL STRINGFIELD

Library of Congress Control Number: 2011908467
ISBN: Hardcover   978-1-4628-9014-9
               Softcover   978-1-4628-9015-6
               Ebook   978-1-4628-9016-3

To order additional copies of this book, contact:
Xlibris Corporation
1-888-795-4274
www.Xlibris.com
Orders@Xlibris.com
96620

CONTENTS

FINDING THE PROBLEM

This is a story of bad doctors and a two-year search for what was wrong with me.

I am better now but may not be alive if I had stayed on the path I was on. Medical practice today is just that, and your life is on the line if your doctor doesn't have enough practice. I think this is very sad and hope that most people have medical practitioners that are not afraid to send you to a specialist out of their medical group.

If anyone that is a doctor reads this book and is offended in the end, I am sorry, but you are just the type I wrote this opening to keep people away from. You are not the smartest guy in the building, and you do not know everything about medicine. The best doctors I know are not afraid to ask. They also don't make snap judgments that could affect the rest of someone's life.

If you don't feel you are getting the medical attention you think you should be getting, say something and hear them out, then make up your mind if you wish to stay with the doctor. The primary doctor I had with the first group was a good, caring doctor; but the other ones—the specialists—were not practicing medicine, they were running blood tests. The bad part of that is that they didn't know what they were looking at on the blood test but the obvious high blood pressure and the like. All the signs of what was wrong with me were in the very first blood test and got worse every time, but he didn't know what he was looking at or didn't care which would be worse.

April 12, 2008. I am not feeling good today when I woke up but didn't think anything of it and got to work. At work, I started feeling worse, but I managed to finish the shift and go back to the apartment and take a pain pill so that I could get some sleep. The pain is always there; it won't go away, but I can block it out most of the time. The longer this goes on, the easier it is to block out the low-level pain. The hard part is when I want to do yard work at home because the pain gets so bad by just mowing the lawn that I need to go inside and lie down after taking a Vicodin for pain.

I am always wondering what it is, and it makes me mad that the doctor cannot figure out what it is. I know I hurt now, but the problem is, I am worried that it will start affecting me at work; and if the inmates think I am in pain all the time, then they will start acting up, thinking that the pain will keep me from doing my job.

This same pain pattern keeps up 'til I go home and go back to the doctor to tell him it is getting worse. Dr. Oh, my primary, really cares; but he is a general practitioner and can only do so much. Dr. Oh does what he thinks is best and sends me to his group's GI specialist.

I will not name this fool because he doesn't deserve to get any credit. The first thing he did was draw blood. Man, there's a new idea. I have had blood drawn every month for the last six months. Dr. Oh had a lower GI run and x-rays with resolution, all along with a CAT scan. None of these showed anything, and that is very upsetting when you know that something is wrong.

Time for another twenty-eight days at work away from the home. Sometimes, I wonder how much the stress of being away from home affects the pain. I can do nothing about it because I have put in for a transfer every year that I have been with the CDC, but they somehow have made it impossible. I had a transfer, but it went to hell when I had the stupid local bank try to make trouble over their inability to follow my instructions when cashing a check. It all turned out the way it should have, but I sure didn't need the hassle. The pain was getting worse, and I could not finish my shift a couple of times and was starting to worry about what was going to happen.

I changed my diet to see if no spicy food will make it go away. Maybe I have damaged my stomach with all the hot food I have been eating. Since Calipatria is only twenty-two or so miles from the Mexico border, you would think that you could get some good Mexican food around this place. That is not the case; it is the same food you get at any chain in LA.

The pain came back in a bad way one day at work, and my supervisor called for an ambulance to take me to the hospital in Brawley. They did an MRI and blood work. They also gave me a shot of morphine that worked very good but doesn't allow for further tests because I don't hurt anymore.

I now have five bottles of painkillers at the apartment. They are the following:

1. Methocarbamol for muscle pain
2. Naproxen for pain, two bottles
3. Hydrocodone/APAP 5/500 (generic for Vicodin), two bottles

Food was the only joy I had when I was down here. The store at the corner of Main Street with the gas pumps was able to make these monster pizzas that were great.

I want to go over what is going on in my mind. Everyone I work with knows I don't feel that good, but they don't say a thing. They know that if the shit hits the fan, I will be there to do what I can, and most of the inmates respond to me because they think I am mean and they know I get even. The average inmate is about sixth-grade level when it comes to education. Most follow really well, so the smarter ones use their brains to control things, and they think they are smart enough for us not to be able to figure out who the shot caller is. It is not easy, but if you watch and they don't know you are watching, then they will give him up. Knowing these people makes your job easier. Some of them will give people up so you will let up on watching them. But you must be alert all the time because they will turn on you in a flash, and most of the time, you won't have a clue.

The best way to work them is with respect. You can use it to get them to let their guard down and talk to you, not just give you a moving mouth.

I tell you all this so you'll understand that my brain is in action as long as I am at work, or your building is going to be out of your control. All this is stress, and I was thinking that this was what was causing my stomach problems. The only problem was that most of the pain attacks came away from work. I started to bring food that was not spicy so as not to upset my stomach. The worst pain attacks came about an hour and a half after work. In every new attack, the pain would get worse than the last one. I worried that I might have an attack that would render me unable to get help.

At work, it was bid time, and you could change jobs if you had enough seniority. I put in for a job in the infirmary to get off the yard. I wanted to see if a job with less stress would make the pain attacks go away. I got the job and had the best partner I had ever worked with. No more shot callers and no more games. Take your meds, and take your dinner. This is third watch from 1400 'til 2200. All the things that were done by the medical personnel were done before third watch.

This job change did make a little difference because I stopped having the pain at work for a couple of months, but I would still have them at the apartment, so I would just take a pain pill and go to sleep. The pain was never there when I woke up in the morning.

I changed doctors when the GI guy said I had stomach cancer, then changed his mind.

The new doctor that I was going to was in Orange County. He was the partner of my wife's doctor, so I felt I was going to the right place, but I never saw the doctor. I only saw his nurse practitioner. She only listened to part of what I told her, but she did set up an upper GI. This came out negative, so she all of a sudden made up her mind that I was crazy and nothing was wrong with me. She went into the check-blood mode every month, and that was it. I told her that I changed doctors to find out what was wrong, and she looked me in the eye and said nothing was wrong, but she did put me on a cholesterol medicine.

The next month, I was fed up and told her I wanted to know what was wrong with me and I had no intention of going through months of blood tests because they did not show the problem.

Her reply to that was to set up a lower GI and take a look. I told her I had a lower GI not six months before, and she said that they might have missed something.

All this just made me mad, but what could I do? I went back to work and, on the third day, had an attack at work and had to leave work. The pain was so bad. My work called first thing the next morning and told me to go home and find out what was wrong and not come back 'til I did.

I went home and talked with my wife about it all and told her that I was going to figure it out. I knew that if I did any hard work or even mowed my lawn, the pain would come.

That night about seven, I had this stabbing pain hit me right in the middle of my gut. My whole body would quake, and the pain would cause me to bend over for any kind of release of the grip the pain had on me. My daughter Dawn saw this and said for me to knock it off or I was going to the emergency room at the local hospital in Pomona.

We headed to the hospital about twenty minutes later and walked into a full waiting room. I told Dawn to take me home because I did not want to wait for hours to get the same old song and dance, but she refused.

Much to my surprise, they called my name about twenty minutes later, and I went over to fill out the paperwork and talk to the ER tech in the booth. I was taken back and put on a bed about ten minutes later and given a shot of morphine. Just what I wanted, but I was starting to like all these painkillers, and that was not a good thing.

They went on to put me in the MRI and took some pictures that told them nothing. The one thing they did that the others didn't is spend about ten minutes talking to me. He told me he could not go any further but that I needed my blood checked because my B was way off and something was wrong.

So now I leave you all with, what do I do now? The pain tells me something is wrong, and this doctor says something is wrong. It is time to come up with a plan, but what kind of plan will get it done?

SETTING UP A PLAN

I have made up my mind that the only way to get to the bottom of what is wrong with me is to go by ambulance with the pain to St. Jude Medical Center in Fullerton and hope I get the right ER doctor.

St. Jude has all the machines they need to find out what is wrong with me. If I get there during normal hours, they even have a full staff of specialists. As of this point, I had no Idea I had cancer—that was the last thing on my mind. I knew something was very wrong, but I didn't even think of cancer.

My youngest girl is coming over to see me, and it won't be nice, but I will make myself sick before she gets to the house and have her take me to St. Jude. All I have to do is mow the front lawn, and that will be enough to bring the pain back. Then all I have to do is get her to take me to the right place.

March 11, 2010. Plan is in motion. I have just finished the lawn, and I hurt like hell, but my little girl is not here yet. My girl Heather is always late. By the time she got to the house, some of the pain had gone away, so I pulled out a bucket and got it ready to wash her car. Finally, she is here, and I tell her we need to wash her car. I get down and start doing the tires, and on the second tire, here comes the pain.

Oh my, I didn't ask for this, did I? Whatever is wrong with me, it does not like me messing around with it. This time the pain has taken over my whole gut, and I dropped to my knees. I tell Heather that we have to go to the hospital, and she grabs her phone to call 911. I tell her, "No, you need to take me to St. Jude in Fullerton and hope I get the right doctor." We get in the car and start for Fullerton. It's about ten or fifteen miles away, but it is the best in the area. We are about three-fourths of the way through Carbon Canyon, almost halfway to the hospital, and I start having chest pain bad. What do I do now? My plan is falling apart, and I wasn't needing anything else to come into the picture. I called the Brea 911 and told them where we were headed and what was happening. They said, "Stay on the phone and stop driving. Our station is around the corner."

The fire truck with the paramedics and an ambulance were coming up from behind us, and they pulled over to the curb, and they opened the door, and I tried to get out but needed help. I was not in good shape by this time. I told them St. Jude, and they said they couldn't code 3 because Placentia-Linda Hospital is closer. I told them what I needed, and we went red lights only to St. Jude. In the ambulance, they gave me something to calm my heart down that helped a little and wanted to give me something for pain, but I would not take it.

We finally arrived at St. Jude, and into the ER, I went. They hooked me all up to the heart monitor and started an IV. The doctor who came up asked me if I was nuts not to go to Placentia-Linda Hospital, and I told him that the heart was okay; and that if I died from a heart attack, then I would not have to worry anymore about what was wrong with me. The doctor and I then talked for about ten minutes, and I told him about what was going on, and he said he would do his best. I didn't know how long I was in the ER, but it was a few hours when the doctor came up and said he had a bed for me and that I should get some rest because I'd have a busy day if he could fit me in. It's 0400 in the morning, and I was awakened to go to the MRI, then to another machine that was supposed to give better detail than the MRI. I think I spent time in every machine they had in the hospital, and they took blood at least four times. No food but two rolls with turkey meat because they did not want food going through my system to mess with the machines. It was about one o'clock on March 13, 2010, and all the testing they could do they did. The doctor said he would talk to me when the family got here. My mind went nuts on that one. Am I going to die, or what the heck is wrong with me that the family needs to be here?

GETTING AN ANSWER

It is about two o'clock when everyone that is coming is here, and I don't like this at all. What can it be? Everyone has a long face, and they are asking me what the doctor said. I don't know anything, I tell them, and they just said I don't have the guts to tell them. The doc walks in, and he introduces himself to my family and says that with all the tests that they have run, they don't see the cause of all the pain. Then he goes on with, "His blood is in bad shape, and it needs to be taken seriously." He would like me to go across the street to the cancer center and see Dr. Park. I asked when, and he said they are waiting. All of us go across the street and Dr. Park's suite at which time I am taken to the back, and Dr. Park says he doesn't know for sure, and he would like a bone marrow sample. I say, "Okay, do we do it here or somewhere?" Dr. Park says right where I am sitting, and that he needs me on my stomach with my pants down. I know it sounds like a joke, but getting your bone marrow taken out is no joke. The pain when they went for the marrow is the worst I felt as if I was bending the table I was lying on.

Everything was happening too fast now. I wanted things to slow down so I could think. Then I would think, *What are you waiting for? You can't get better thinking. Just keep it together enough to know when you are getting better.* The doctor says that it will take about three days for all the tests to be run, and he will call us then.

We all go out to dinner and then home and bed. I am beaten and need to sleep in my bed, which I did very well all night. I woke up at 6:00 am, got dressed, and took my grandson to school. He asked if I was going to pick him up, and I said I didn't know, the doctor might call. Most of the day, I just rested and looked up the cancers of the blood. This was not a smart thing to do because I didn't need most of the information. About 1:00 pm, the phone rang, and it was Dr. Park, asking me if could I be at his office asap. I said yes, then got on the phone and called everyone. We all arrived at the doctor's about the same time, and in we went. I felt like a race driver waiting for the start of the race. Time has stopped, and it won't move. We all headed upstairs to Dr. Park's suite, we checked in, and I paid my first $15 c/o pay.

The nurse came out and got me and my wife and the one daughter who came along. He laid it on the line and said that I had AML, but that he wanted to stain the cancer cells to make them easier to count and then I might have an anemia and not leukemia. He said to go home and relax and that it would take about three days before he would have us back when he gets the results.

The next day, he called and asked if we could be there and then asked if we could be there at the same time. I responded with a yes. I called who needed to be called and then headed for Park's office. I was farther away than anyone that I called. My brain had been running at five hundred plus miles an hour and wouldn't slow until we know for sure. I never hope so much for a low count, but even then I would think I am not that lucky. This is not funny. I wanted something you could cut out and rest awhile, then go back to work. As I drive through the canyon, I think about what this all means—maybe a little "Why me?" or a whole lot of "Why me? Why me?" is not productive. And by the time I got to his parking structure, I saw that everyone was there. We all went upstairs and checked in at Dr. Park's office. They were waiting for us, and my brain just quit the game and went on to what was next. We all went into the same room as before, and Dr. Park was standing there with no smile. My brain just shut down. I did not want to hear what was next because I would have to accept something I don't want to accept.

He went on to explain what a blast cell was and again said that under 20 percent was not classified as *cancer*. Then he again went over the way they stained the cells, and only the blast cells turned colors. Then he looked at me and said my blast count was thirty-nine and that I needed chemo as soon as possible. I said, "Okay, let's go and do it," thinking he couldn't get me in right away, and that would give me time to make sure I was right with God and allowed my mind to absorb the news.

Dr. Park said he needed to check and left the room. We all looked at one another, and one of my girls asked, "Why so fast, Dad?" I tried to sound brave and told her why. Let it sit on your mind and make you crazy, which is probably what it would have done. They had a room, and I told the family to bring my pj's because I had no intention of looking like a sick person any longer than I could. I got a "Dad, you will look like a sick person because you are one, and your pajamas won't make it change." I told them it would help keep my mind in the right place, and I needed all the help I could get.

STARTING DOWN THE LONG ROAD

We all went across the street to the hospital to the room on the cancer floor that they told us to go to. Everything for the rest of the night was a blur. It didn't matter where I was because I was playing the "Why Me" song in my head over and over. I knew more than I wanted about AML—acute myelogenous leukemia. It is caused mainly by working around benzene, which has not been on the market since I was a young man working around it at my dad's plant. The only problem with that idea is that the cancer normally shows up within five to six years of exposure and that work with Dad was thirty years ago.

They came in within fifteen minutes of the time they put me in a bed with the chemo. One big bag of clear stuff that runs for twenty-two hours, and a little orange one that runs for three hours. No problem. Let's get the show on the road. They also gave me a Benadryl to relax me. The orange stuff hit me like a truck, and I rolled over on my side, went into the fetal position, and went to sleep. As I started to go out, I prayed for God's help in my waking up. They woke me up at six in the morning to have a glass of juice and a fist full of pills, then said I would be going for a ride for a bunch of tests at seven. Off I went at seven for a CAT scan, and an MRI was supposed to be done until the guy saw me, and I said, "Do we really need two of these in three days? I am going to glow in the dark." He laughed, then made a couple of calls, and back to the room, I went. I felt good that morning, but I didn't want to see the orange stuff again, and I knew I had two more days on it and four more days on the clear. It's funny how I never wanted to know the name of any of the chemo drugs. I just felt it was too much information and didn't want to know. Now I should have asked so I could tell you all, but it would scare you all to death if you ever had chemo. I think this way is best. Just be ready for whatever comes and hold on. None of them are meant to be nice. They are going in you to kill the cancer and not to kill you. I think they have tested all of them, so they are not meant to kill you. You have to keep in mind that the cancer is now part of you and will take over, and this is not what you want. You would be unable to keep going.

Next day is the same as the first, except there was no ride downstairs for anything. The orange stuff was meaner this time, or I was a little weaker from the first day. All I knew was that I don't like this stuff and it sure as hell doesn't like me. You can feel it going into your system, and you know you are in for a hard run. Every day I would take something to help me sleep through it because I knew I would get sick if I stayed awake while this stuff ran through my system. I did get to sleep, but when I woke up, I felt like it had taken everything I had, and my guts just rumbled, wanting to throw up but holding it back. My wife, Cheryl, showed up after work. She was just what I needed at that time—someone to hold my hand and try to make me feel better. It is crazy how something so small can make you feel better. It was as if I was getting energy from her hand, but I really did feel better. I think it's just having someone you love with you at a time that you really need a loved one.

The third day was the worst. I just knew this stuff was eating the life out of me, and I could feel it going away. I didn't know what to do, so I went to God for the help I needed, and I felt better after praying the whole time that the orange was going in. I had, since that day, been much stronger in my faith, but I still had a long way to go that I would learn before it was all over. I had two more days of this chemo, but it was just the clear one, and that stuff didn't bother me at all. I didn't feel right for weeks and, to this day, have not felt as good as I did before it all started. One chemo down and three to go. But at this stage of the game, I didn't know I had three to go. All I knew was that this one was over and that I get to go home before the next one. I was not going home until I recover from this, and they would come in every morning and take blood to check the cell count, and they would release me when the count was high enough. This took about two weeks, then I got to finally get out of the hospital.

I went to my Michelle's house to stay because she was a nurse, and everyone figured that was the best place. She has two little ones, and we all had a blast. Even though I did not have a lot of energy, my grandson and I would play 'til Papa was gassed; then I would lie down and take a nap, and they would go on with their normal life as best as they could with me around. Just going up and down the stairs in her house would kick my butt. I would go down to eat or play with the kids and would have to sit down and rest before we could play. I now know why young people have kids and us old ones just go to visit. A one-year-old boy can burn you out in no time, but it was great while it lasted.

I was back for more chemo in two weeks; this one seemed to go a lot better, and I didn't feel anywhere near as sick while I was getting it. I had an easier time being in the hospital. Also, I had mentally adjusted to being in bed most of the day. I had also brought my laptop and was on Facebook almost all the time. I hate to say it, but Facebook made the time in the hospital go by a lot faster because my mind had something to do. I played every game they had at that time because I would get bored playing the same game. Also, Facebook made it so I wasn't so mental about what was going on with my treatments. At six o'clock every morning, they were in taking blood and then they would bring in what they called a meal. All of it was good for me, but with the chemo, the taste buds did not work right, and most of the food had no taste. It is no fun no matter what you have to do to have to go through this sort of thing.

I did not realize how important it was to have visitors every day. How the human contact that was not a hospital worker would help put your mind at ease. My family was great at coming to see me. My wife, Cheryl, and daughter Dawn came by almost every day; and the other kids made it at least once a week. This was great, and I didn't realize how important it was until I went to City of Hope for my stem cells. Being alone most of the time, even with Facebook, was hard on me. I am a people person and do not like being alone. Most weeks at City of Hope, I would go four or five days without any human contact but staff; and no matter how kind they are, it just is not the same.

I did not go home this time. I stayed until chemo three. What a joy, they didn't want me to overdo it, so they just kept me on ice until I could handle chemo three. It was not as bad as three and seven, but it was not as easy as the second one they gave me. My stomach was upset all the time, and I did not want to eat. All the food tasted the same—bad. The chemo had killed my taste buds, so the only flavors I got were bad and horrible. How do you eat to keep up your strength if everything you eat tastes bad? You eat because you don't want the monster inside you to win. Most of the time when I eat, it would try to come back up, and I would send it back until it stayed. I know that every person reading this just felt sick. Try that feeling for twenty-four hours a day for weeks on end. This is why I think many people give up and let the cancer win. They get sick and tired of being sick and tired and don't know any other way but to quit. God will give you the strength to survive if you ask. You may have to pray many more hours than normal, but this is a big job, and the attack is always going on, so don't stop praying. You have to stay strong to help God help you. I am not sitting here writing this without doing it. I prayed like I have never prayed in my life. I was not ready to leave this life even if the next one is better than what they say it is. I still have time to do good deeds, and I want the option to do some. I want to go back to the hospitals that I was at and talk to the people and try to get them to ask God for the help they need, or give them this book and have them read it and hope that it helps. You do not have the strength to do this fight on your own; you need a higher power. If you do not want to accept God, then please look for something else to go to that will give you help. Have someone in the hospital come and talk to you so you have a better understanding of what God means in all our lives. If you get a person of a religion you don't like, then ask for someone else. If you know you want an MS Lutheran and you are in a Catholic hospital, just ask. They will understand and call someone to come in and see you. I was taking prayers from everybody that came by to give them because I figured they couldn't hurt. My God is not a different God than somebody else's, we just follow in a little different way. All the good books in the many churches say the same thing, but in a way that they want you to follow. Ask for a Bible, and someone will bring you one. It can't hurt, and I might be right and it will help.

This is not a fight that any of us wanted to fight how we got it if they knew they could stop cancer but they don't know or are not saying because they are not sure. In any case, it all boils down to "You got it, and now you have to fight it." I assure you, none of us wanted it.

Somehow, I have managed to only lose a few pounds because I kept shoving the food down, knowing and being told that I needed the strength that the food supplied. I finally made it home but was to go back to St. Jude in two weeks for a prep chemo for the stem cells I will be getting. The two weeks turned into three days, and I would only see home for about four days before I go to City of Hope. I was given an IV with blood platelets the first two days, then some other stuff—for what, I don't know—but it made me feel better, and I started walking around every day in an attempt to keep my legs working as best as they could. All the chemo had taken its toll on me, and I could only do about four trips around the unit before I got tired and got back in bed. The nurses and a couple of the nurse helpers would come by and talk every day, and that made the days go faster. Most days, I would get a visitor or two, and that would help out a lot at keeping me from thinking about what was going on.

I got to go home after about two weeks because I was to go to City of Hope for some tests and meet Dr. O'Donnell, the best doctor I have ever known. At first I thought she was a tough one because on the first visit, she asked a lot of questions and went over some things, then was gone. Her nurse practitioner went over the timing of everything and asked if we had any questions, then went over the papers to see that everything was filled out, then told us that I would be going back to St. Jude for a prep chemo for the stem cells.

My memory was bad before I got sick, and it is wasted now. If I am thinking right this time, home my oldest daughter took on a new husband. The wedding was at our church, and I got a new suit and gave her away like all good fathers do. What a day. I don't know where all the energy came from. After the wedding, we went to my sister's house for the reception. I had a great time but started to feel a little burned-out and found a place to sit down and take it all in that way. By the time it was over, I was completely burned-out and happy it was over so I could go home and rest.

I was back in St. Jude after three days at home and now would not go home but for a very busy week before going into City of Hope for my stem cell transplant. It was to be done in about a week to ten days when Dr. Park came in and asked if I could wait a month because someone needed stem cells right away, and they wanted to use my spot in time. I told him that would be fine as long as it didn't affect my health. That was when he told me that I was in remission and that I had nothing to worry about. He would be watching me.

I spent another month in St. Jude with the same daily blood tests and an IV of antibiotics and water going in my arm. I asked him why I was getting so much water, and he said it was to keep me hydrated. At the beginning of week three, they started an IV that was part of the prep for the stem cells. He called it prep, but it kicked my butt. I was on the toilet ten times a day, and it seemed that as soon as I got back in bed, I needed to go again. I would still get my walks in because that seemed to settle things down. At the beginning of the last week, I had a new nurse come in my room at night to remove an IV line. She did it really fast, and all I wanted to do was go to sleep. Something woke me up a few minutes later, and I reached up to rub my head because it always calmed me down. My eyes were still shut, but I was awake. I felt something wet on my head after I had rubbed it. I opened my eyes to see blood on my hand and looked at the spot where the IV was, and it was bleeding. I am good around other people's blood; I have never been good around my blood. I don't want to see it, and when I do, I tend to get very light-headed. When I saw the blood, I pushed the nurse button and waited for what seemed like a long time. I then got out of bed and went to the nurse station for help because I needed them to stop the bleeding. It wasn't bleeding that bad, but it was not supposed to be bleeding at all. I was talking to the nurse in charge when I felt light-headed, and that is the last thing I remember 'til I felt someone hit me in the chest and yell, "Mr. Stringfield, breathe." I could not get my eyes to open, and I couldn't hear any more sounds. Then everything came on, and I opened my eyes to see a room full of staff looking at me and the charge nurse rubbing my head, saying, "Don't do that again, you scared the hell out of us." Then she said that when I went down, I stopped breathing, and they called a code blue, and that was why all the people were in the room.

I couldn't think straight, so all this information was just going in and not being handled right. My brain was still in a fog, and it stayed that way for about ten more minutes. She came back in after everyone had left and told me that I could not get out of bed without a nurse being present and that meant going to the bathroom also. I still don't know why that happened, except to say that I think it was all the stress and then the blood on my arm was the frosting on the cake. I don't know, but I did what they said because they told me if I started having problems, I may not get my stem cells because I am sixty-one and City of Hope doesn't want any problems.

I still worked out a way to get my walks in, and they relaxed a little on the escort. On many mornings, they would come in just to see how strong I was so that when I went for my walk, I wouldn't fall down and cause a problem. When you are 6 feet tall and 220 plus pounds, having you fall out is not good because it takes most of the staff to get you back in bed. I didn't want to go down any more than they did, so when I felt bad, I would stay in bed. On those days, they would come in and see what was wrong and do what they could to make me feel better.

I didn't know until much later that Dr. O'Donnell was told about it and almost cut me off. She told Dr. Park to have me come to City of Hope on a given day for a battery of tests, and that would tell her if she wanted to take the risk.

If I had not gotten the stem cells, I would have gotten chemo every time the cancer came back; and from what I have been told, even though I was in remission, it would come back. And if they didn't catch it in time, I would be gone.

That means going to Dr. Park all the time for them to check my blood and see if there are any signs of the AML returning, and if so, another bone marrow sample and another round of chemo is needed.
THE TRIP TO CITY OF HOPE

I made it through all the tests with flying colors and was sent back to St. Jude for one last trip to get a chemo for the stem cells. This stuff was not nice. This is a direct attack on your blood, and it lays you out and stomps on you. It wasn't like the others that made you feel sick to your stomach. It made your whole body feel like it was slowly being killed. You could feel your energy and your strength being drained from you. You are slowly dying, and it is on purpose. All you can do is *pray* and *pray* some more and hope with all your hope that God hears your prayers. I thought I was as low as I could go and still get up. No more walks, just the TV, and MacBook kept me from going nuts. My visitors kept coming, and everyone was told that I was going to win this fight. The only change was that I was starting to question about what was next, and wondering if I had what it would take to get through it.

I thought that I had been praying up 'til now, but I had just begun. I asked the Lord to forgive me for all my sins and forgive me for my weakness and failure to spread his love and understanding to all the people that I touch. I will never go a day for the rest of my life and not thank the Lord for what he has done for me. I will not go and talk with anyone without bringing God into the conversation. I will be his loving servant for the rest of my life.

I said these things and did not have any idea that I would be back, asking for the same thing again before it was all over. I meant everything I said the first time and meant it even more the next time.

I stayed in the hospital for a week after that nasty stuff and went home on a Friday. All my kids and most of my grandkids were over that night, and the ones that were not there were at the house before the weekend was over. I have a very loving family, and hopefully, my girls will all continue that for the rest of their lives.

Monday—off to City of Hope for an infusion that takes about two hours. On this day, it is a little longer because my wife and I get to meet with Dr. O'Donnell. We repeat the infusion Tuesday, Wednesday, and Thursday; then we pack up on Thursday night because I am going back to the hospital on Friday and getting my stem cells on Wednesday.

Friday morning arrives with a feeling of doom. I know the stem cells are the hot stuff now, but I don't want to go back in the hospital. Somehow, I knew that this was not going to be the six-week stay they are talking about. The IV they give you on Friday is the worst thing that has ever been put in my body. It took all I had to keep from losing everything I ate for the next two days. The next two days are for recovery from the Friday bag and to build you back up for Monday's bag. Oh my God, I prayed all day Monday, asking that he give me the strength to survive this stuff that is being put into me. Now was another one of those times in the whole treatment that you eat to stay alive, not because you want to. Nothing tastes any good, so you have to try everything to see what you can handle. Most things you can eat have to be cooked, and some of the stuff, you still cannot have because it grew up under the dirt and not on top. Strange enough, but you can have onions as long as they are grilled onions. Oh heck, no, I don't want any grilled onion on my burger. I love grilled onions on my burgers. You had to be careful with it because some of the cooks have no idea of how to grill an onion, so when they are on duty, you do not order a burger. With all the things that were happening every day to help you get better and the chemo brain you have to work with, all this stuff is hard to do. Sometimes my brain was so out of sync, I would just sit there in bed and want to cry. This could not happen because I am a sixty-two-year-old male, and I don't break down and cry. I was a prison guard, a truck driver, and a few other things in my life; and to break down and cry would be a violation of my image. But violation or not, it happens at times when everything would pile up and there was nothing I could do about it. I would curl up in my bed with my back to the door, and let it go. I was never caught doing this, and now I am telling you about it because it would release stress, and that was good. I have always held this type of thing in because my dad would tell me men didn't cry. This emotion was locked up, and at sixty-two, it was only the third time that it had gotten out since I was in my teens. Don't be afraid to let your emotions out, and if a good cry is what you need, just let it go. I don't know why, but you always feel better when it is over. So let it happen. It drains some of the stress off, and you'll sleep like a baby.

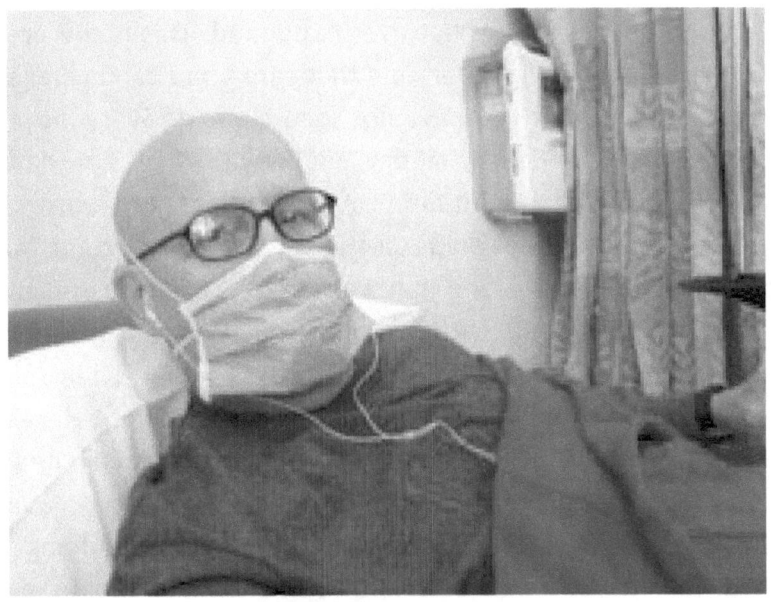

It's been six weeks plus in the hospital at City of Hope. Long days except on the weekends, and they were way too short. I got most of my visits on the weekend unlike at St. Jude where I had visitors almost every day. City of Hope was not just over the hill. It was about thirty-five miles from the house through some of Los Angeles's worst traffic. So most of the family couldn't come during the week. It was asking too much of them to make that drive to visit someone with chemo brain. I say chemo brain as a reason because we cannot follow a very detailed conversation. I looked forward to the weekend because I got a lot of visitors and it kept my mind off why I was in there in the first place. During the week, they would all call and ask how I was, and I would say fine no matter how I felt. No need to make them worry until someone could come and see my face. They didn't ask how I was, they could all tell by looking at my face. If it looked bad, they would lie and say how good I looked, and it would help me feel better, but most of the time I felt better just having visitors. On those days, I slept better because having the visitors would wear me out and make going to sleep that much easier. When you are in bed all day long and on most days get at least a one-hour nap, most of the time it is hard to get to sleep.

Facebook is the best thing that ever happened. This is the greatest way to keep in touch with everyone that cares. You can even keep in touch with people that you have not seen in years. Every morning, I would post how I was doing that day, but I wouldn't say how bad I felt if even if I was feeling bad. I didn't want the family to worry about me all day long until they could call and see what was wrong. I would say it was not a good day, and that was it. Some of those not so good days were not good at all. Those were the ones where I questioned if I could win the fight, how much weaker could I get, and if I could still put up a worthwhile fight. If my stomach got upset, it was hell because that was where the GVH was, and it would make me feel all the sicker. I couldn't fool any one of the medical people because they could see my face, and they all knew what it looked like when I was doing good. I had learned how to order food that would help, and that food thing worked out very good. A lot of the time if I had some soup, it would settle things down, and I would start to feel better. Back to Facebook. I would spend hours every day on the farms or cafe or whatever doing my work. It was great because it took my mind off what was going on and kept me busy playing the games. All my people would send me messages to keep my spirits up, and it worked. It worked because for that split second, I would not be thinking about me. I had someone who had gone through what I have gone through, tell me not to worry about things I might forget. If you want to remember it, you have to write it down and put in everything about it because you will forget all about it. That is very true in many cases, but in a few, it is not. The few are very few, like what time do I pick up my buddy from school? I pretty much have that part down to "He only has to tell me when the time changes, like every Friday, it seems they get out early." If he doesn't tell me, I will forget and show up at the normal time. All this is something that makes me mad at myself but then I just get grumpy, and everyone pays.

The food here was much better than the other hospital because you ordered what you wanted to eat, and in most cases, you would get it just how you asked. Even these people made sure that you didn't eat anything that you were not supposed to.

I didn't want to die, but I was afraid of what life was going to be like after I got back out of the hospital. No one sat down to say what I could do or could not do until the day I got out. I thought the world of my doctor. She is the best, but she would just say to not worry about it, "You have to fight to get well enough to go home." She was right, of course, but you still want to know. She did take the time, on the day I finally got to go home, to tell me what I could do for the next year. *Nothing*.

STEM CELLS

My stem cell donor lives in Northern Italy and was a twenty-one-point match. A ten-point match is good enough to transplant into someone else. The donor center at City of Hope said they were going to send him more family questions because he has got to be related to me. They told me this the day before, so I start thinking this is going to be a walk in the park. *Wrong, wrong, wrong*. This has been anything but a walk in the park, but my time since transplant has been much easier than most. You don't know who this person is, but you do know the sex and the age. My partner and roommate at work is also sick with AML and is at KIASER Hospital getting his chemo. I won't go into details for his privacy. As bad as I thought I had it through the whole process compared to his was a walk in the park. He has gone through hell and will finally get his stem cells thirty-eight days from my writing this. We talk about every two weeks, and I make him feel better. I pray for him every day and ask God to help him on his road to post-stem cells. I tell him to relax, he is coming to City of Hope for his transplant, and to keep eating. Everything will be all right.

Back to my donor. He is thirty-eight years old and male. He calls the donor center all the time to see how I am doing, and he will be coming to the United States some time in late August after the year is up, and he knows who I am. This is all they will tell me about him, and that is all he knows about me. This is to not cause him great pain if I don't live that long. They took one million stem cells from him and sent them for me. They put half a million stem cells in me, so I have a full dose as backup for a year. They are no good after that for anyone. It seems like a waste of good stem cells, but in most cases, if something goes wrong, they have to find a new donor or go back to the original if it has been long enough.

Graft-versus-host disease is what they call the interaction between the two sets of stem cells. They are not going to get along. Yours will fight the donor cells, and the donor stem cells will fight back. Your cells have had their butt kicked by the chemo, so you would think that it wouldn't be much of a fight. The closer the match, the less of this goes on because as in my case, I think they don't see them as bad guys. I am not saying

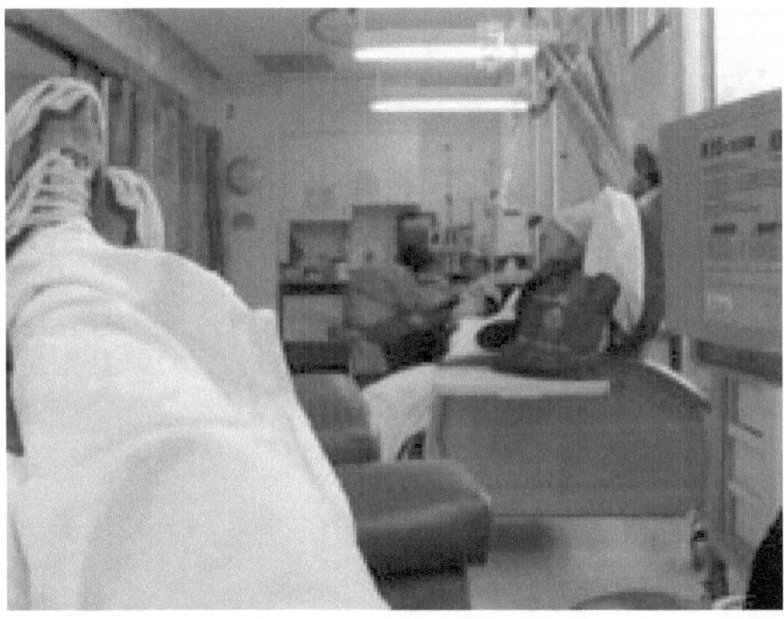

that I have not had any GVHD, but it has not been as bad or lasted that long. As I write this, it is March 2, 2011, and I received my stem cells on August 18, 2010. This is not a very long time as stem cell battles go. I have met people at the hospital that got their stem cells over five years ago and still have a lot of trouble with the GVHD. My GVHD settled in my digestive tract and was raising hell the day after they went in. The pain that I had prior to them finding the cancer was in the same place, so this is not that bad, and it makes it a lot easier to handle.

Every day, no matter how I felt, I would go for a walk because I always felt better after the walk. It was a 16th of a mile around the whole building. I would walk a minimum of thirty-two laps in the morning, and if I felt really good, I would do it again in the afternoon. This always made me feel better because it would get my blood flowing better, and that always helped. I would stop and talk to anyone that would listen because being in the room alone was not that much fun when you had already spent months in the hospital. At St. Jude, I could get an aid to stay and talk with me, but at City of Hope they all were too busy, and the nurse would chase them down.

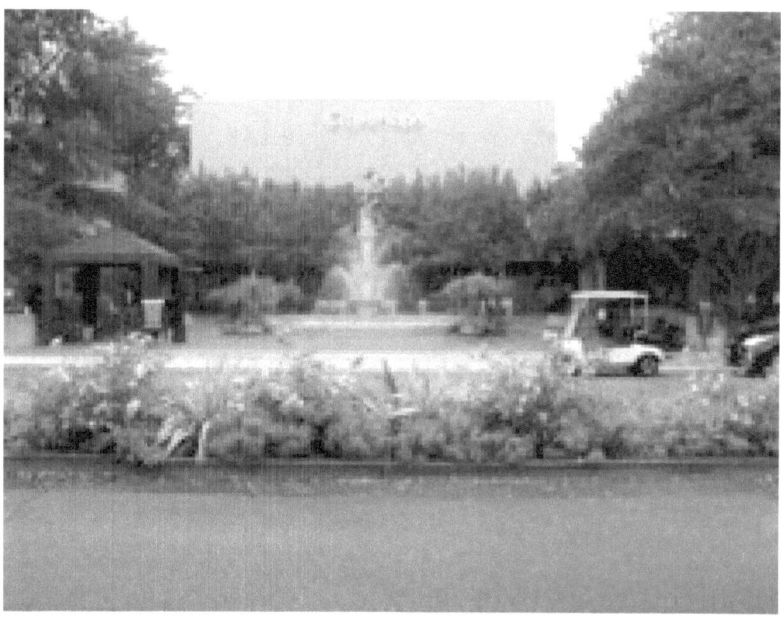

Some mornings, I would wake up to the pain and stay in bed a little longer but would always get up and walk because it made me feel better and made the pain go away. When the pain was there, my mind would go wild with the thoughts of doom. I was tired of hurting and wanted it to go away for good, but I didn't know at that time that it would be months to come, and for many people that get stem cells, it never goes away. If I had known this at that time, I don't know how I would have held up. The pain is from the stem cell battle going on inside of you, and it is just something you have to deal with. I now can block most of it out because it never gets as bad as it was. Every day, you win a little more ground in the battle to have your health back. Even though it gets in your mind and you want to give up so, it will all end. I would get like this and start to pray to my Lord to help me keep my mind clear and help me with the pain. Some days I would walk, and it would get worse. On these days, I would not walk in the afternoon. I would stay in bed and pray.

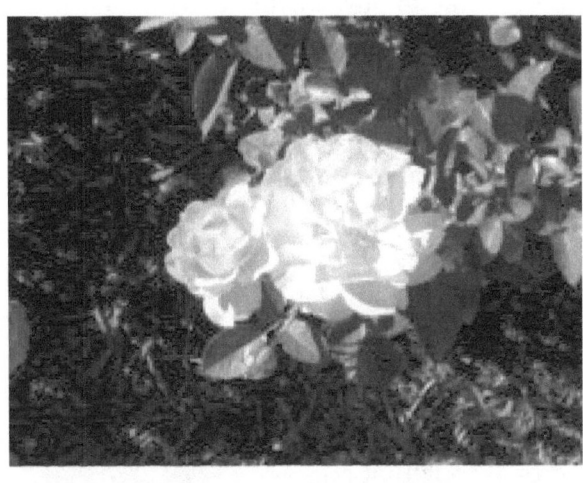

My pastor was great. He would come and see me almost every week, and we would pray. This helped me keep my mind in a good place, but the pain would always come back. On this one day, I was hurting bad and praying for him to give me a sign that this was a good fight that I needed to keep up. I must have said the right thing that morning because the spirit of the Lord came into my room, and the room was bright with light even though no one had touched a light. I was in no pain, and my mind was clear. My Lord and Savior Jesus Christ was in the room, letting me know that this was a good fight and that he needed me here on earth. I was not done with the work he wanted me to do. He let me know that this was a good fight and that I could fight it and would come out okay. While this was going on, Pastor D came into the room for a visit, and I sat up and said, "Can you see it? Jesus is here, the room is all bright." But it wasn't to him. We talked about what was going on and then prayed to the Lord. He was with me all this time and stayed for a while after Pastor D had left.

I went for my walk about an hour later and told some of the nurses, but I think they thought I was nuts. All they would say was, "That was nice," and go about what they were doing. The charge nurse came to my room to talk to me. I think she wanted to determine if I had lost my mind, but when she left the room, she was no longer thinking I was crazy. The pain was there, but now it didn't matter and I knew I was in the right place and was soon released from the hospital. I did not go home I wet to stay in the apartments they had on the grounds for people that did not need to be in the hospital but needed to have daily medical treatments and could not be more than thirty-five minutes from the hospital. I spent the next 45 days in the apartment walking into the hospital and getting an IV and blood draw, chasing away CVM. This is a hospital virus that I had picked up at St. Jude that needed to be gotten rid of. It took that long because the top two treatments for getting rid of a virus caused a reaction in me, so I was 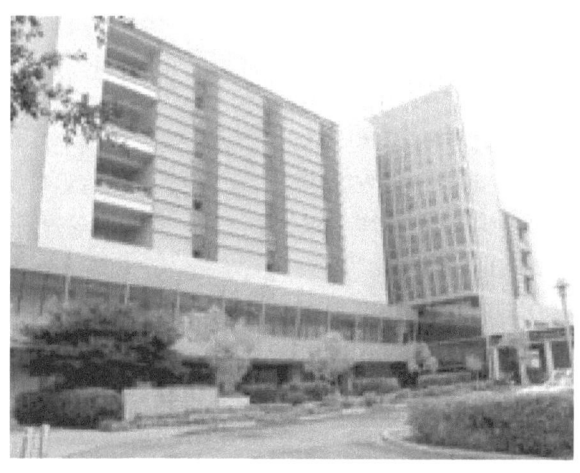 unable to have them. To this day, I wear an allergy bracelet around my wrist.

The apartment was crazy because I could not be there alone, so the whole family had to come together and pick a day to stay with me. The good part was that I spent quality time with everyone and ate good food as long as it met the standards set out by Dr. O. The list was not that limiting, and they had a Trader Joe's only about a mile away. I could come and go as I wanted as long as I spent the night in the apartment and didn't miss my daily IV. I saw Dr. O every Monday and Thursday and also had a blood draw on those days. I had a PICC line in my right arm, so this was never a matter of new holes in me every day. Both

hospitals put in PICC lines, but St. Jude never used the one they put in, so in one of the times between chemos, I had them take it out. I kept the one in my arm from City of Hope for about two months after the daily IVs had stopped. That was just my

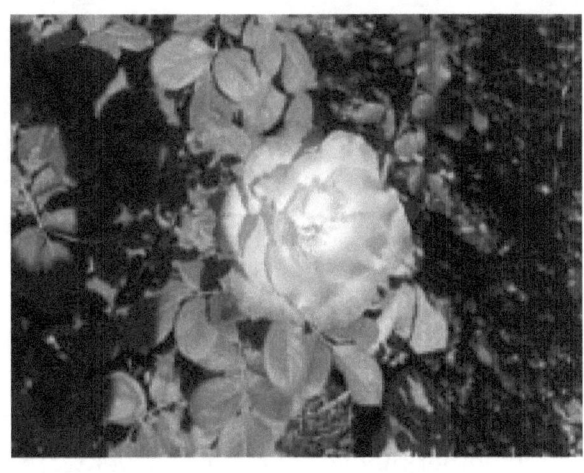

worrying that I would get sick, and they would need it. I now have twenty-one bottles of pills that I take at least once a day and some as much as three times a day. Many of these are steroids that are meant to keep the stem cells under control. Some of these are the vitamins that I have always taken, but it is a lot of medication to deal with. The

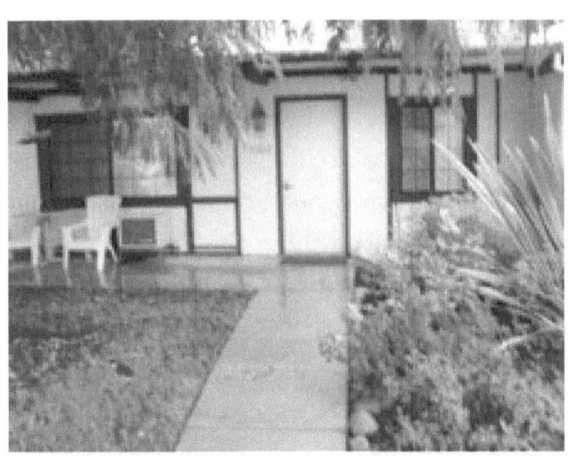

old saying of "being sick and tired of being sick and tired" is now in effect. Chemo brain is your brain being affected by all the drugs that you have taken. At this point in time, it is still there. It is now from all the pills, and the wife and family will just shake their heads when I say something that doesn't fit the moment. Nothing you say now comes automatically. You have to think about what you want to say, then think about if it is the right thing to say. Much of the

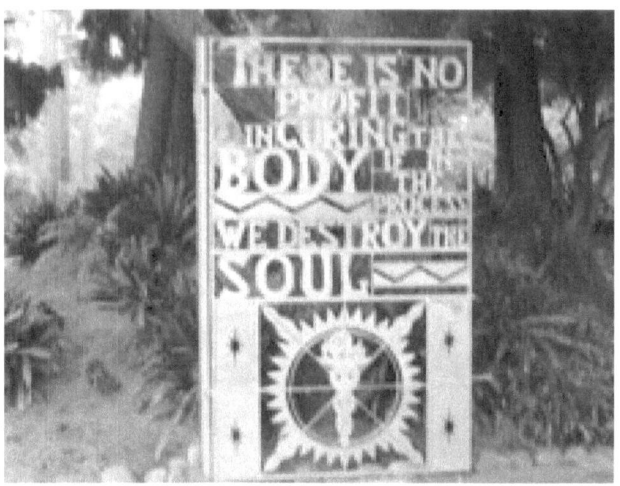

time, it is just better to keep your dumb mouth shut. It drives me crazy at times when all my girls are around and talking because I cannot mentally keep up. Then they always say, "What do you think, Dad?" and I just say, "Don't ask me. You figure it out and let me know what is happening." You have to remember that your brain will never work the way it did before.

Many of the things you did before will come back to you automatically, but driving the car is not one of those things. You know the rules, and you know how to drive, but you get mad at the other drivers easily. You don't understand what is going through the mind of the idiot. This normally happens to a much greater degree than it ever did before you got sick. How many people have almost spun out a car with front-wheel drive? Well, I did on a dry road, and if it wasn't for the front-wheel drive, it would have gone all the way around. I don't even know how I did it, but I do know that I do not want to do it again. The other thing wrong with that is it gets your blood flowing, and you have to lie down and rest when you get home. Another little thing they don't tell you until you ask. Your energy level is a blip. You can do things at a slow pace, or don't do it at all because the meds you are on have taken most of your energy.

Some of these things were getting chalked up as my being out of shape, and it will get better. I don't think it will because every time I extend myself, it takes the same amount of time to start feeling the way I did before I did it. I love my yard, and I like working in my yard. I get great pleasure when I have no weeds in my front yard planters, where I grow daylilies and irises. With all the time I was in the hospital, the planters are full of weeds, and I don't have the energy to get rid of them in one day. I am two weeks into working in the front yard, and just now I am getting ready to go after the weeds. I should have flowers by late April, so I need to hurry up at the pace I am going. This whole cancer thing, even seven months after transplant, is messing with my every goal. This, I am told, I have to live with, and it will get better in time after I finish taking the cancer meds. So I ask Dr. O when I will stop taking the cancer meds. She smiles her sweet smile and tells me the day after I die if I follow her instructions. Stem cell transplant patients never stop taking the meds.

I have not worked in nearly a year and have managed to stay even with the house payments and utilities. Everyone else has had to sit back and hope we get money from somewhere extra to pay them. The ones that got nasty about it have not seen any money since they opened their big mouth. It doesn't bother me one bit, but I didn't know my wife was doing it until just a short time ago. With my brain, you wouldn't give me the checkbook at all. I have learned to go to the store with just a little money.

I want to go to work, but Dr. O says she will think about it in October 2011, not before then, so don't bother her about it. I don't know what I can do, but there must be something. I have no energy, so it cannot be a physical or high-energy type of job. I can only work in the yard for about thirty minutes and then I am wiped out for the rest of the day. This is something that all new cancer patients must come to grips with. The pills you take for the rest of your life are going to limit your ability to do many of the things you did before you became ill. This thing is not a joke, and at times, I wonder if the ones that lost the fight are not the lucky ones. That being said, I will fight on to do the best I can to live as normal of a life as I can. Dr. O says that if I do what I am told, there is no reason that I won't live into my eighties. Now that is old to me, and it means that if I am good, I have another eighteen years of life in this world. That means that I can see all my grandkids through high school and many of them through college. As the old saying goes, "You have to live your life to the fullest." I am doing that to the best of my ability, but so many things need to be done that I did before that I am unable to do now. My wife says to act my age, but I have never acted my age, so why start now? As time goes by, I find out what I am unable to do or at least do in the manner that I did them before.

THE LOOK

Only a sick person would notice this. I am 6 feet tall and I am still 220 lbs. In the hospital and up until two months ago, I was over 240 and did not at all look like a sick person. Dr. O would not let me lose weight. She said that this was what made me able to fight all the side effects of the chemo and the pills. Again I say you have to eat all your meals, and they have to be meals, not snacks, to fight this. It will kick your butt if you give it a chance.

The people around you are always watching what you are doing and how you do it. Many of them are loved ones, and they care very much about how you feel. Your brain is not working right because of all the drugs that are running through your body. You say stupid things because that is what comes out of your mouth. You didn't mean to say it the way it came out, but your brain is not working right, and that is the way it came out. This is when you get the look from others. They will start giving you the look before you even open your mouth after awhile. I have started to not say things off the cuff because that always comes out wrong. I don't understand this at all because I can sit here and write this and then read it back, and it all looks right to me. All of my thought is fragmented and come to me in small bursts. That is what you are reading, and this is how your brain works on the meds. I hope I made this clear. I am writing it first thing in the morning before the brain is fogged up like it gets at night. You are not stupid, and the important things that you would think about anyway seem to go okay, but when people are giving you a lot of information and handing you things and someone else is trying to help explain, your brain overloads and you get all the details messed up. Most of the time, I will tell people to write it down so I can read it; then I will let them know. The pills you get when you go home from the hospital the last time are the pills you will spend the rest of your life taking. When I first left City of Hope, I was taking forty-two pills a day. They would have you so torn up, all you would do was walk or sit in front of the TV. Please take note that I didn't say watch TV. I would watch sporting events and things like that, but if there's anything that had a speaker sitting there talking about something, I would turn the channel because I couldn't follow along. Only about half of his story would remain in your head and that half did not make any sense. First thing in the morning, you could get up and watch the news and get it. If you don't take a nap, then the longer you stay up and the harder it is to retain anything you were told. The more pain you are in will affect what you retain, but I think that would be for anyone. Years ago I wrecked a motorcycle and was in unreal pain, and today, I cannot bring those days back, it is all blank. I only remember a couple of things during that time.

It is funny how things work. I had a laptop with me all the time I was in the hospital and would post how things were going with my chemo and stem cells. I would try to post somewhat positive things so I wouldn't have my phone ringing off the hook from family. I love them all dearly, but they can drive you nuts if they are worried about you. Being a loved one meant the worry was already there, but bad news would take it to new level. Most of the time, they read the message and could tell when I was making light of my status. They would call the hospital and talk to the nurse on duty before they would talk to me. Then they would talk to me and give a hard time because I was not telling them the truth. I told them that they couldn't do anything to help, so why have them worry all day until they get off work? Once I was at City of Hope, I would get mad at the nurse if she made them worry because on workdays it just wasn't a drive that I wanted them to make. How in the world can you make your family relax with all that is going on? My wife would come visit and hold my hand for most of the time that she was there. The only time that she didn't was when I was feeling bad, and all I wanted to do was sleep. It is not normal to sleep as many hours as I did when I didn't feel good, but it was the only way to get through it.

You looked forward to when the stem cells came and then found out that they caused pain too. Is this what life had in store for me for the rest of my life—fighting pain? As it turned out, this was not the way it was. The longer the stem cells were in me, the easier it was. You still have little pains here and there but not something that is worth talking about, and in time, you can block them out with your mind.

As I write this, it has been almost one year since it all started. It is March 10, 2011, and my first chemo was started on March 24, 2010. The memories are still strong, but the hard times are not seeming so hard. This next week, I get another bone marrow test to see if the cancer is still in remission. The thirty-four pills I take every day are with me for the rest of my life. They are my lifeline, and without them, they don't know what will happen. Maybe the stem cells won't kill me if I stop, but it is not worth the risk. The little energy I have would be better without the pills, but it is not worth the risk. Once you have blood cancer, your life is changed forever. Good or bad, that is the way it is.

I go to the hospital and see people that have been in remission for years, and the GVHD is kicking their ass. Graft-versus-host disease is with them for the whole time since the transplant of stem cells. The drugs are meant to control this, and the better the match, the less trouble you have. My match could not have been better than it was every way they looked at it we matched. Because of that, I have had a minimum of problems. The only time they act up is when I eat something that is too spicy. That is because my stem cells, or I should say my GVHD, is in my digestive tract, so I get a gut ache like never before.

My last six weeks at City of Hope were in the apartments on the property for patients that don't need to be in the hospital any more but need to stay within thirty minutes of the hospital in case something goes wrong. These places cost you sixty-five dollars a day like a hotel, but you have no room service, and someone in the family has to stay with you so that if anything happens, they can call for help. Look at the pictures that I end the book with, and you will see how nice it is and how well the grounds are kept up. My wife and I would go for walks every night for our health, and the grounds would help us with our peace of mind.

The rose bushes were coming in to bloom just before I went home. I am not a rose lover, but I do like to walk in the rose garden at City of Hope; it is too nice to pass up. This is where I began to heal. I knew I would not have seen this if I was not going home soon. I would walk in the park and rose garden every chance I had because it would be the first time in many months that I could stop thinking about what I had been going through.

My praying to God made the long months go by with peace of mind and soul. This would not be possible if I did not believe. You need someone to help with the pain and help carry the load, and God is and was the only answer I had, and it worked. I hope you read this and understand where I am coming from in this battle against cancer.

THE START OF A NEW LIFE

This new life is full of new daily things that I must do to stay alive. Counting my vitamins, I take thirty-nine pills a day, thirty-two of which are because of the cancer, leaving only seven as vitamins. Steroids, I always thought, were for freaks that wanted bigger muscles than what their body could make. Also, I knew of some that were taken after an injury or surgery where muscles were involved to aid in the healing and return to normal movement. Now I know of four that are taken after a stem cell transplant to help control the graft-versus-host disease, this being the battle between your stem cells and the new ones that are donated by some wonderful person that wants to help sick people live a better life and win the battle against cancer. The steroids have made me diabetic, and this is no fun. I am injecting insulin into myself four times a day and my whole life up 'til I got sick. I was the type that would get weak at the sight of a needle. I hate this part of my new life because it has caused more of a change in how I do things than anything else. Every morning, I wake up to check my blood sugar and then inject some insulin. If I am going some place that may take more than a couple of hours, I need to pack some snacks and all my diabetes supplies up and take them with me. I know people that are diabetic and have never seen them doing this stuff. I have a friend that only takes his insulin after he eats. I take mine, then I eat, so I still have a lot to learn.

I have had to give up my job because the doctor has told me that I am unable to return to that type of work. I don't know what is going to happen because I have no energy, and it will only improve a little. Nobody goes through this and goes back to a physical labor or high-energy type of job. My partner at work has now gotten his stem cells and is doing fine, but he keeps saying he is going back. He might get back, but it will be to a desk job, and he will still be around a lot of people at work, and I have been told that this is not the type of environment that we can go back to. But he has different doctors, and they have not told him a thing.

I am sixty-two years old and have filed for social security, and I am trying to get disability from my job because I have enough time in to qualify. For my whole life, I have enjoyed working in my yard and making it look nice. Now I have to hire people to do things because I just don't have the energy to do it. If you push yourself, you can do some of it but nowhere near what you could do before you got sick. If you do push yourself, you will be weak for two days after that, and I was told that this is not to be done.

I will have to adjust how I think about the yard and make it so it doesn't need that much work. If you know someone who is out of the hospital from blood cancer and has had stem cells transplanted, go over and help them if you have the time. They will not want you to out of pride, but let them complain and help them out. I am now a housekeeper, a yard keeper, and a head cook in my house; and it takes everything I have and some help to get things done. I am lucky because I am out of the hospital and doing great, but the adjustments that need to be done in your life are many, and if you don't, you end up back in the hospital.

I have cheated the grim reaper once and hope that I don't have to fight him off again. I don't want to go back into the hospital. I have been in there for too long, and it is too hard on me.

I am back to Saturday men's Bible study and church every Sunday that I am not feeling bad, but I still miss some because you just don't feel good every day. Before I got sick, I would have one of those off days, but you go ahead and do what you want because you know it will go away. Now I have to shut down and take it easy, or it will mess up many more days. The "feeling bad" now is, your body just feels worn-out from the minute you wake up, and you cannot eat anything that will change or drink an energy drink to get you going because the energy you use will not be available the next day, and it will put you down for a few days while getting back to normal. Life is to be enjoyed now. I don't think about the fact that this thing could come back, and I would have to go through the whole thing over again. "I am cured" is the only way to think. I must get on with my life even if I cannot go to work. I will get social security and a pension from my old job. The pension will only be about 1,200 dollars, but that is better than just Social Security, and all my medical needs will be paid for, so life is not too bad.

My whole family got together the other night to go to dinner because it had been one year since they told me I had AML, and the doctor told the family—not me—that I only had a 20 to 30 percent chance of making it. Sure am glad no one said that to me. I just don't know how that would have gone over. My mind may have not been that much into the fight. I don't know. It was a good fight, and I am still alive, so I am stronger than the doctor thought. Praise God for helping me be strong enough to get through something I didn't know had the odds against me. My family didn't tell me that until the dinner the other night, and I am thankful for that.

If you have a loved one that is going in for treatment be brave for them. They need your help to get through this and if you are all upset and show it they will know and it will make it a much harder fight. If you go to church ask God for the power to fight the decease. If you don't go to church you need to find a higher power then yourself to help you through this.

I pray daily for God to give strength to all sick people. Don't be afraid to ask God he is listening and he will help.

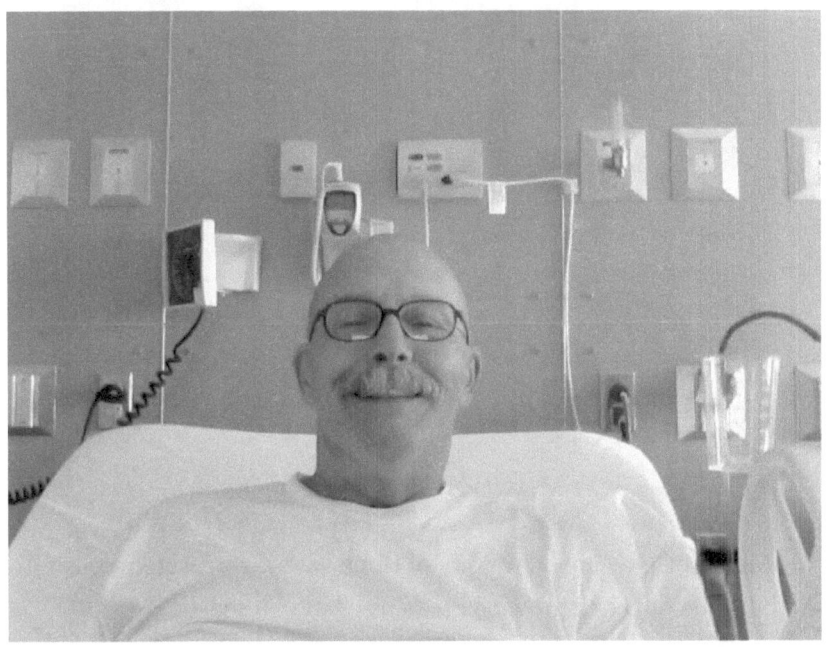

At St. Jude after 3 of the chemo waiting to go home

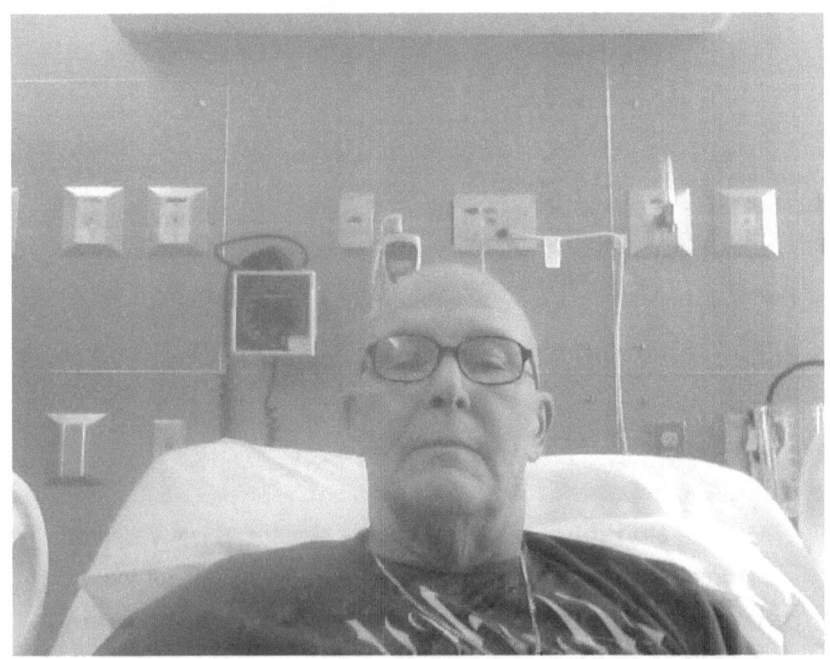

All the chemo is done and all the hair on my body is gone

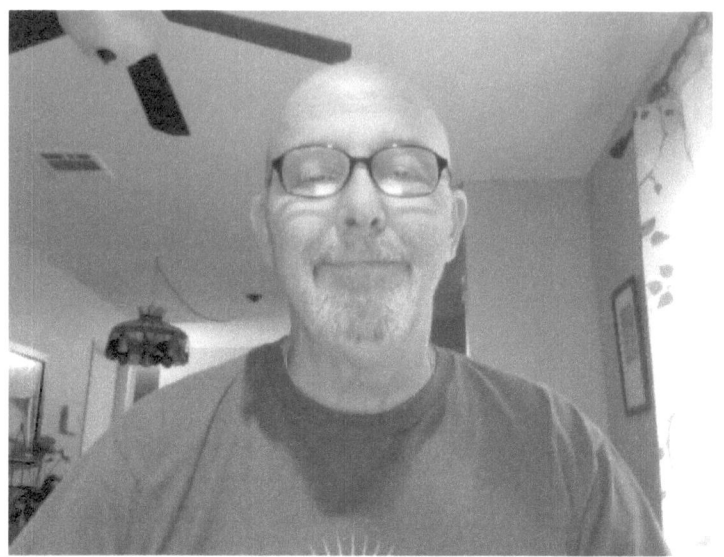

Start of a new life out of City of Hope with my new stem cells and the only hair growing on me is what you see.

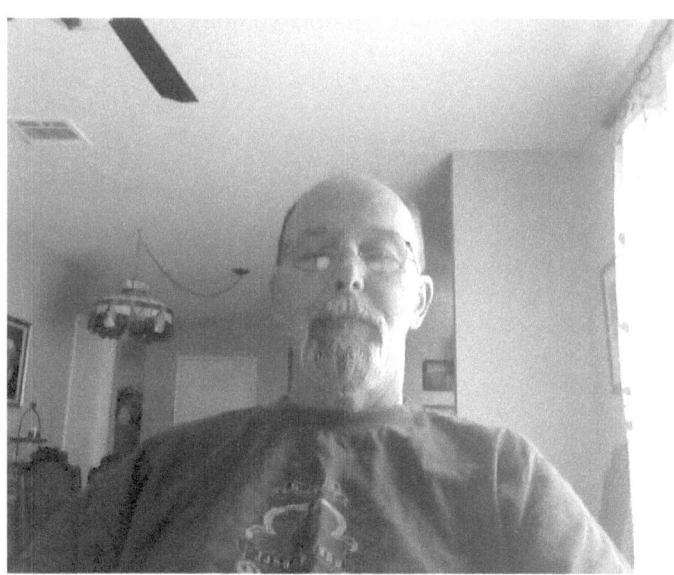

May 20, 2011 the gotee is not going anyplace. It is my sign of completion. I am not as mean as the thing makes me look. I have most of the hair back that is coming back. The drugs are strong and make you a mental toy for other people. You have to sit back hear it all out then respond to what they said.

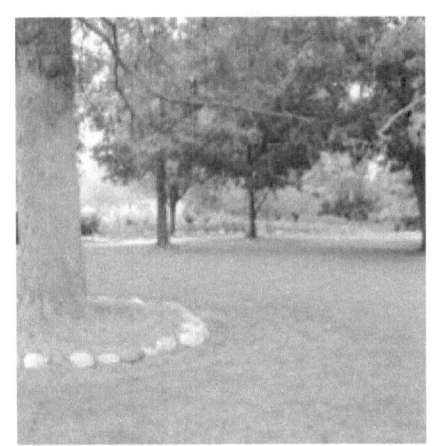

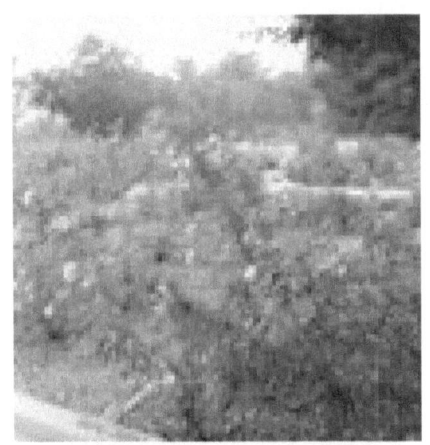

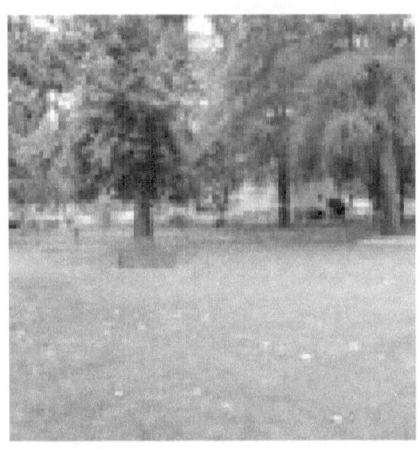